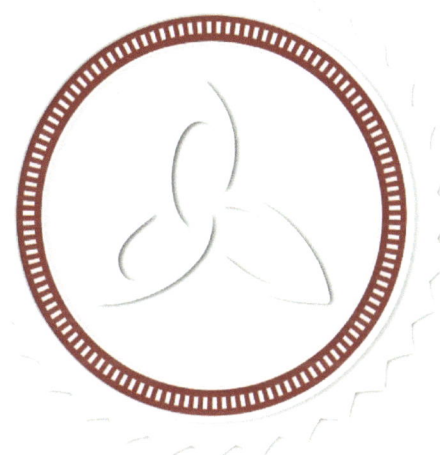

Trinity Fitness

By Jackson John-Maire

Food Plan

Trinity Fitness

By Jackson John-Maire

Disclaimer & Disclosure

Trinity Fitness

By Jackson John-Maire

Healthy eating tips: Set yourself up for success

To set yourself up for success, think about planning a healthy diet as a number of small, manageable steps rather than one big drastic change. If you approach the changes gradually and with commitment, you will have a healthy diet sooner than you think.

- *Simplify.* Instead of being overly concerned with counting calories or measuring portion sizes, think of your diet in terms of color, variety, and freshness. This way it should be easier to make healthy choices. Focus on finding foods you love and easy recipes that incorporate a few fresh ingredients. Gradually, your diet will become healthier and more delicious.
- *Start slow and make changes to your eating habits over time*. Trying to make your diet healthy overnight isn't realistic or smart. Changing everything at once usually leads to cheating or giving up on your new eating plan. Make small steps, like adding a salad (full of different color vegetables) to your diet once a day or switching from butter to olive oil when cooking. As your small changes become habit, you can continue to add more healthy choices to your diet.
- *Focus on how you feel after eating*. This will help foster healthy new habits and tastes. The more healthy food you eat, the better you'll feel after a meal. The more junk food you eat, the more likely you are to feel uncomfortable, nauseous, or drained of energy.
- Every change you make to improve your diet matters. You don't have to be perfect and you don't have to completely eliminate foods you enjoy to have a healthy diet. The long term goal is to feel good, have more energy, and reduce the risk of cancer and disease. Don't let your missteps derail you—every healthy food choice you make counts.

Trinity Fitness

By Jackson John-Maire

- *Try not to think of certain foods as "off-limits."* When you ban certain foods or food groups, it is natural to want those foods more, and then feel like a failure if you give in to temptation. If you are drawn towards sweet, salty, or unhealthy foods, start by reducing portion sizes and not eating them as often. If the rest of your diet is healthy, eating a burger and fries once a week probably won't have too much of a detrimental effect on your health. Eating junk food just once a month will have even less of an impact. As you reduce your intake of unhealthy foods, you may find yourself craving them less or thinking of them as only occasional indulgences.

- *Think smaller portions.* Serving sizes have ballooned recently, particularly in restaurants. When dining out, choose a starter instead of an entree, split a dish with a friend, and don't order supersized anything. At home, use smaller plates, think about serving sizes in realistic terms, and start small. If you don't feel satisfied at the end of a meal, try adding more leafy green vegetables or rounding off the meal with fresh fruit. Visual cues can help with portion sizes-your serving of meat, fish, or chicken should be the size of a deck of cards and half a cup of mashed potato, rice, or pasta is about the size of a traditional light bulb.

Trinity Fitness

By Jackson John-Maire

- *Listen to your body.* Ask yourself if you are really hungry, or have a glass of water to see if you are thirsty instead of hungry. During a meal, stop eating before you feel full. It actually takes a few minutes for your brain to tell your body that it has had enough food, so eat slowly.

- *Eat breakfast, and eat smaller meals throughout the day.* A healthy breakfast can jump-start your metabolism, and eating small, healthy meals throughout the day (rather than the standard three large meals) keeps your energy up and your metabolism going.

- *Avoid eating at night.* Try to eat dinner earlier in the day and then fast for 14-16 hours until breakfast the next morning. Early studies suggest that this simple dietary adjust-ment—eating only when you're most active and giving your digestive system a long break each day—may help to regulate weight. After-dinner snacks tend to be high in fat and calories so are best avoided, anyway.

Trinity Fitness
By Jackson John-Maire

- *Greens*. Branch out beyond bright and dark green lettuce. Kale, mustard greens, broccoli, and Chinese cabbage are just a few of the options—all packed with calcium, magnesium, iron, potassium, zinc, and vitamins A, C, E, and K.
- *Sweet vegetables*. Naturally sweet vegetables—such as corn, carrots, beets, sweet potatoes, yams, onions, and squash—add healthy sweetness to your meals and reduce your cravings for other sweets.
- *Fruit*. Fruit is a tasty, satisfying way to fill up on fiber, vitamins, and antioxidants. Berries are cancer-fighting, apples provide fiber, oranges and mangos offer vitamin C, and so on.

Trinity Fitness
By Jackson John-Maire

Eat more healthy carbs and whole grains

Choose healthy carbohydrates and fiber sources, especially whole grains, for long lasting energy. In addition to being delicious and satisfying, whole grains are rich in phytochemicals and antioxidants, which help to protect against coronary heart disease, certain cancers, and diabetes. Studies have shown people who eat more whole grains tend to have a healthier heart.

A quick definition of healthy carbs and unhealthy carbs

Healthy carbs (sometimes known as good carbs) include whole grains, beans, fruits, and vegetables. Healthy carbs are digested slowly, helping you feel full longer and keeping blood sugar and insulin levels stable.

Unhealthy carbs (or bad carbs) are foods such as white flour, refined sugar, and white rice that have been stripped of all bran, fiber, and nutrients. Unhealthy carbs digest quickly and cause spikes in blood sugar levels and energy.

Tips for eating more healthy carbs

- Include a variety of whole grains in your healthy diet, including whole wheat, brown rice, millet, quinoa, and barley. Experiment with different grains to find your favorites.
- Make sure you're really getting whole grains. Be aware that the words stone-ground, multi-grain, 100% wheat, or bran can be deceptive. Look for the words " whole grain" or " 100% whole wheat" at the beginning of the ingredient list. In the U.S., Canada, and some other countries, check for the Whole Grain Stamps that distinguish between partial whole grain and 100% whole grain.
- Try mixing grains as a first step to switching to whole grains. If whole grains like brown rice and whole wheat pasta don't sound good at first, start by mixing what you normally use with the whole grains. You can gradually increase the whole grain to 100%.

Avoid: Refined foods such as breads, pastas, and breakfast cereals that are not whole grain.

Trinity Fitness

By Jackson John-Maire

Enjoy healthy fats & avoid unhealthy fats

Good sources of healthy fat are needed to nourish your brain, heart, and cells, as well as your hair, skin, and nails. Foods rich in certain omega-3 fats called EPA and DHA are particularly important and can reduce cardiovascular disease, improve your mood, and help prevent dementia.

Add to your healthy diet:

- *Monounsaturated fats*, from plant oils like canola oil, peanut oil, and olive oil, as well as avocados, nuts (like almonds, hazelnuts, and pecans), and seeds (such as pumpkin, sesame).

- *Polyunsaturated fats*, including Omega-3 and Omega-6 fatty acids, found in fatty fish such as salmon, herring, mackerel, anchovies, sardines, and some cold water fish oil supplements. Other sources of polyunsaturated fats are unheated sunflower, corn, soybean, flaxseed oils, and walnuts.

Reduce or eliminate from your diet:

- *Saturated fats*, found primarily in animal sources including red meat and whole milk dairy products.

- *Trans fats*, found in vegetable shortenings, some margarines, crackers, candies, cookies, snack foods, fried foods, baked goods, and other processed foods made with partially hydrogenated vegetable oils.

Trinity Fitness

By Jackson John-Maire

What is a healthy daily limit for saturated fat and trans fat?

Experts recommend you limit the amount of saturated fats you eat to less than 7 percent of total daily calories. That means, for example, if you need about 2,000 calories a day, no more than 140 of them should come from saturated fats. That's about 16 grams of saturated fat a day.

No more than 20 of those calories should come from transfat. That's less than 2 grams of transfat a day. Given the amount of naturally occurring transfat you probably eat every day, this leaves virtually no room at all for industrially manufactured transfat.

Source: American Heart Association

Trinity Fitness
By Jackson John-Maire

Put protein in perspective

Protein gives us the energy to get up and go—and keep going. Protein in food is broken down into the 20 amino acids that are the body's basic building blocks for growth and energy, and essential for maintaining cells, tissues, and organs. While too much protein can be harmful to people with kidney disease, the latest research suggests that most of us need more high-quality protein than the current dietary recommendations. It also suggests that we need more protein as we age to maintain physical function.

How much protein do you need?

Protein needs are based on weight rather than calorie intake. Adults should eat at least 0.5g – 0.8g of lean, high-quality protein per kilogram (2.2lb) of body weight per day. A higher intake may help to lower your risk for obesity, osteoporosis, type 2 diabetes, and stroke.

- Older adults should aim for 1 to 1.5 grams of lean protein for each kilogram of weight. This translates to 68 to 102g of protein per day for a person weighing 150 lbs.
- Divide your protein intake equally among meals.
- Nursing women need about 20 grams more high-quality protein a day than they did before pregnancy to support milk production.

Source: Environmental Nutrition

Trinity Fitness
By Jackson John-Maire

Limit sugar and salt

If you succeed in planning your diet around fiber-rich fruits, vegetables, whole grains, lean protein, and good fats, you may find yourself naturally cutting back on foods that can get in the way of your healthy diet—sugar and salt.

Sugar

Sugar causes energy ups and downs and can add to health and weight problems. Unfortunately, reducing the amount of candy, cakes, and desserts we eat is only part of the solution. Often you may not even be aware of the amount of sugar you're consuming each day. Large amounts of added sugar can be hidden in foods such as bread, canned soups and vegetables, pasta sauce, margarine, instant mashed potatoes, frozen dinners, fast food, soy sauce, and ketchup. Here are some tips:

- *Avoid sugary drinks.* One 12-oz soda has about 10 teaspoons of sugar in it, more than the daily recommended limit! Try sparkling water with lemon or a splash of fruit juice.

- *Sweeten foods yourself.* Buy unsweetened iced tea, plain yogurt, or unflavored oatmeal, for example, and add sweetener (or fruit) yourself. You're likely to add far less sweetener than the manufacturer would have.

- *Eat naturally sweet food* such as fruit, peppers, or natural peanut butter to satisfy your sweet tooth. Keep these foods handy instead of candy or cookies.

Trinity Fitness
By Jackson John-Maire

How sugar is hidden on food labels:

Cane sugar or maple syrup

Corn sweetener or corn syrup

Honey or molasses

Brown rice syrup

Crystallized or evaporated cane juice

Fruit juice concentrates, such as apple or pear

Maltodextrin or dextrin

Dextrose, Fructose, Glucose, Maltose, or Sucrose

Trinity Fitness
By Jackson John-Maire

Salt

Most of us consume too much salt in our diets. Eating too much salt can cause high blood pressure and lead to other health problems. Try to limit sodium intake to 1,500 to 2,300 mg per day, the equivalent of one teaspoon of salt.

- Avoid processed or pre-packaged foods. Processed foods like canned soups or frozen dinners contain hidden sodium that quickly surpasses the recommended limit.
- Be careful when eating out. Most restaurant and fast food meals are loaded with sodium. Some offer lower-sodium choices or you can ask for your meal to be made without salt. Most gravy and sauces are loaded with salt, so ask for it to be served on the side.
- Opt for fresh or frozen vegetables instead of canned vegetables.
- Cut back on salty snacks such as potato chips, nuts, and pretzels.
- Check labels and choose low-salt or reduced-sodium products, including breakfast cereals.
- Slowly reduce the salt in your diet to give your taste buds time to adjust.

Trinity Fitness
By Jackson John-Maire

Bulk up on fiber

Eating foods high in dietary fiber can help you stay regular, lower your risk for heart disease, stroke, and diabetes, and help you lose weight. Depending on your age and gender, nutrition experts recommend you eat at least 21 to 38 grams of fiber per day for optimal health. Many of us aren't eating half that amount.

- In general, the more natural and unprocessed the food, the higher it is in fiber.
- Good sources of fiber include whole grains, wheat cereals, barley, oatmeal, beans, nuts, vegetables such as carrots, celery, and tomatoes, and fruits such as apples, berries, citrus fruits, and pears—more good reasons to add more fruit and vegetables to your diet.
- There is no fiber in meat, dairy, or sugar. Refined or "white" foods, such as white bread, white rice, and pastries, have had all or most of their fiber removed.
- An easy way to add more fiber to your diet is to start your day with a whole grain cereal, such as Fiber-One or All-Bran, or by adding unprocessed wheat bran to your favorite cereal.

How fiber can help you lose weight

Since fiber stays in the stomach longer than other foods, the feeling of fullness will stay with you much longer, helping you eat less. Eating plenty of fiber can also move fat through your digestive system at a faster rate so that less of it can be absorbed. And when you fill up on high-fiber foods, you'll also have more energy for exercising.

Trinity Fitness

By Jackson John-Maire

Snacks

Trinity Fitness
By Jackson John-Maire

Healthy Trail Mix

Ingredients

- 0.5 ounces unsalted whole wheat pretzels
- 1.0 tablespoons walnuts
- 1.0 tablespoons sliced almonds
- 1.5 tablespoons raisins

Directions

1. Combine pretzels, raisins, walnuts and almonds. Serve.

Healthy Cucumber Snack

Ingredients

- 0.5 cups cucumbers sliced
- 4.0 tablespoons hummus
- 16.0 reduced-fat crackers I use Wheat Thins
- 0.25 cups green olives sliced

Directions

1. Slice cucumber and green olives up.

2. Spread a little bit of hummus on each cracker.

3. Top with cucumber and green olives.

4. Multiply ingredients for more people as an appetizer.

Trinity Fitness
By Jackson John-Maire

Carrots and Raisins (Healthy Snack)

Ingredients

- 2.0 large carrots
- 0.25 cups raisins
- 3.0 tablespoons sour cream
- 2.0 teaspoons sugar

Directions

1. Place raisins in a small amount of water, so they plump up a little. (this step is optional) Grate carrots on a smallest part of your grater.

2. Combine grated carrots, sour cream, raisins (take them out of water prior) and then add sugar (adjust to your taste).

3. We love it just the way it is and my l'il one gets his nutrition.

4. Beware, this combination may make your kids grow few inches taller. Carotene with sour cream and sugar is a dangerous mix for your kid's growth potential.

Trinity Fitness

By Jackson John-Maire

BreakFirst

Trinity Fitness
By Jackson John-Maire

Oat bran-Banana Breakfast for One

Ingredients

- 0.5 bananas chopped
- 0.333 cups oat bran
- 1.0 dashes salt
- 0.75 cups water
- 1.0 teaspoons sugar or honey

Directions

1. Combine chopped banana, oat bran, salt, water and sugar (use more or less sugar to taste) in a microwave-safe bowl.

2. Microwave on high for 3 minutes, stirring after each minute.

3. If using honey, stir it in after cooking.

4. If desired, serve with milk.

Trinity Fitness
By Jackson John-Maire

Blueberry Blast Breakfast Smoothie

Ingredients

- 0.667 cups frozen blueberries
- 0.667 cups fresh blueberries
- 0.5 cups vanilla yogurt can use fat free
- 1.0 bananas
- 0.5 cups fruit juice your choice we use blueberry, raspberry or white grape juice
- 1.0 tablespoons wheat germ

Directions

1. Put ingredients in a food processor or blender and pulse until it is your desired consistency.

2. For a thicker shake or if you use fresh berries add a few ice cubes.

Trinity Fitness
By Jackson John-Maire

Big Breakfast Cookie

Ingredients

- 0.333 cups oatmeal
- 1.0 tablespoons raisins
- 1.0 tablespoons flour
- 0.333 cups non-fat powdered milk
- 0.25 cups applesauce
- 0.25 teaspoons cinnamon
- 0.25 teaspoons baking powder
- 1.0 tablespoons Splenda granular

Directions

1. Preheat oven to 350°F.

2. Spray cookie sheet with baking spray.

3. Mix all ingredients together.

4. Spoon 1 large mound on the baking sheet.

5. Bake 15-20 minutes.

Trinity Fitness
By Jackson John-Maire

Peanut Butter Banana Breakfast Smoothie

Ingredients

- 1.0 bananas cut into chunks
- 1.0 teaspoons peanut butter
- 3.0 ice cubes
- 0.5 cups skim milk
- 0.5 cups soymilk

Directions

1. Puree the frozen banana in a blender, processing for about 30 seconds.

2. Add the peanut butter, process again.

3. Now add the ice cubes, and process until some of them are crushed.

4. Finally, add the milk, process until smooth and pour into a tall glass to drink.

Trinity Fitness
By Jackson John-Maire

Breakfast on an English Muffin

Ingredients

- 4.0 English muffins cut in half
- 8.0 crumpets cut in half
- 0.333 cups peanut butter
- 0.333 cups honey
- 2.0 bananas thinly sliced
- 0.125 teaspoons cinnamon

Directions

1. Preheat grill (broiler).

2. Lightly toast muffins or crumpets.

3. Spread peanut butter evenly over muffins or crumpets.

4. Spread honey evenly over muffins or crumpets.

5. Top with bananas.

6. Place on oven tray under grill (broiler) until honey starts to sizzle.

7. Sprinkle with cinnamon.

Trinity Fitness
By Jackson John-Maire

Vegan Oatmeal Pancakes

Ingredients

- 0.333 cups quick oats
- 0.333 cups water
- 2.0 teaspoons sugar
- 0.5 teaspoons baking powder
- 0.5 teaspoons cinnamon
- 1.0 dashes salt

Directions

1. Grind oats using a blender into a flour.

2. take the oat flour and put it in a bowl, mix in the cinnamon, baking powder, salt, and sugar. Then add the water (you can use milk or soy milk, rice milk, whatever). Now is the time to add in extras like extracts.

3. Mix until well combined, lumps are OK.

4. If your using any kind of fruit gently fold in,.

5. Heat a griddle and spoon out some of the mixture, let cook until bubbles appear and pop at the surface and it will lift without falling apart.

6. Gently flip and let throughly cook through about 1-2 minutes.

7. Keep warm.

8. YUMMY!.

Trinity Fitness
By Jackson John-Maire

Super Healthy Strawberry & Blueberry Smoothie

Ingredients

- 0.5 cups soymilk regular milk works too
- 0.5 cups blueberries fresh or frozen
- 1.0 cups strawberries fresh or frozen
- 6.0 ounces non-fat vanilla yogurt any flavor will work

Directions

1. Blend all ingredients in a blender until smooth and enjoy!

Trinity Fitness
By Jackson John-Maire

Paleo Breakfast Veggie Hash With Eggs

Ingredients

- 1.0 tablespoons extra virgin olive oil
- 2.0 tablespoons butter
- 2.0 garlic cloves minced
- 0.25 cups sweet white onions chopped
- 1.0 cups yellow squash chopped
- 0.5 cups mushrooms sliced
- 1.0 to taste salt and pepper
- 1.0 cups cherry tomatoes halved
- 1.0 cups fresh spinach chopped
- 4.0 eggs poached or cooked any style

Directions

1. Heat large non-stick skillet over medium heat. Add olive oil and butter to pan. Add garlic and onion and saute for 2 minutes, then add chopped squash or your favorite vegetable, cook for 2 more minutes, then add mushrooms. Cook for 5-minutes or until almost compete.

2. At this point add salt and pepper, then add tomatoes and spinach and cook until spinach wilts. Drain well before plating.

3. While finishing this prepare eggs to your liking (I like over medium as this is easiest) in another pan.

4. To serve, drained hash mixture to and then add to individual plates. On top of hash add 2 cooked eggs per person.

5. This is nice served with a side of bacon, and some avocado.

Trinity Fitness
By Jackson John-Maire

Healthy Omelet on the Run

Ingredients

- 0.5 cups egg whites I use eggbeaters
- 1.0 teaspoons onions finely minced
- 1.0 mushrooms chopped
- 0.25 cups spinach chopped about 12 leaves
- 1.0 tablespoons low-fat cheese shredded
- 1.0 to taste pepper to taste

Directions

1. Mix all in very large mug and microwave for 3 (I have a low watt microwave you may need more or less time depending on your microwave).

Trinity Fitness

By Jackson John-Maire

Lunch

Trinity Fitness
By Jackson John-Maire

Broccoli and Apple Salad

Ingredients

- 2.0 tablespoons sugar
- 6.0 tablespoons apple cider vinegar
- 2.0 tablespoons Dijon mustard
- 1.0 tablespoons canola oil
- 0.5 teaspoons fresh ground black pepper
- 1.0 dashes salt
- 1.0 heads fresh broccoli coarsley chopped
- 0.5 lbs apples chopped Fugi or Braeburn are best
- 0.25 cups sweet onions finely chopped

Directions

1. In large bowl, whisk together sugar through salt. Add broccoli, toss well. Add apples and onion, toss again.

2. Cover, chill at least 4 hours.

Trinity Fitness
By Jackson John-Maire

Chicken, Mango, and Rice Salad

Ingredients

- 1.5 cups uncooked rice preferably short grain
- 1.333 lbs boneless skinless chicken breasts
- 2.0 tablespoons oil
- 1.25 teaspoons salt
- 0.75 teaspoons fresh ground pepper
- 0.75 cups red onions
- 1.0 mangoes peeled and cut into 1/2 inch dice
- 1.0 Avocados peeled and cut into 1/2 inch dice
- 3.5 tablespoons lime juice about 2 limes
- 0.75 cups cilantro

Directions

1. Cook rice until done, and rinse with cold water.

2. Coat chicken with 1 tbs. of the oil and season with 1/4 teaspoons of the S/P.

3. Cook chicken until done.

4. When chicken is cool enough to handle, dice into 1/2-inch pieces.

5. Toss the rice, chicken, onion, mango, avocado, and rest of the oil (1 tbs), remaining salt and pepper, lime juice, and cilantro.

6. Chill for at least 1 hour before serving.

7. Revision: Since posting this recipe, I have been trying to cut back on consuming empty carbohydrates. So when I make this now I use little to no rice, and fill it with more of the other ingredients. It is still very good, especially after marinating for a while.

Trinity Fitness
By Jackson John-Maire

Turkish Salad

Ingredients

- 1.5 cups tomatoes
- 1.0 cups green bell peppers
- 1.0 cups cucumbers
- 0.5 cups fresh parsley
- 0.333 cups green onions
- 0.25 cups fresh lemon juice
- 2.0 tablespoons water
- 1.0 tablespoons olive oil
- 0.25 teaspoons salt
- 0.125 teaspoons fresh ground pepper

Directions

1. Combine all ingredients in a bowl and chill for at least 1 hour before serving.

Trinity Fitness
By Jackson John-Maire

Guacamole Salad (Barefoot Contessa) Ina Garten

Ingredients

- 1.0 pints grape tomatoes halved
- 1.0 yellow bell peppers seeded and 1/2-inch diced
- 15.0 ounces black beans rinsed and drained
- 0.5 cups red onions
- 2.0 tablespoons jalapeno peppers seeded 2 peppers
- 0.5 teaspoons lime zest
- 0.25 cups lime juice 2 limes
- 0.25 cups olive oil
- 1.0 teaspoons kosher salt
- 0.5 teaspoons fresh ground black pepper
- 0.5 teaspoons garlic
- 0.25 teaspoons ground cayenne pepper
- 2.0 Hass avocadoes seeded, peeled, and 1/2-inch diced

Directions

1. Place the tomatoes, yellow pepper, black beans, red onion, jalapeño peppers, and lime zest in a large bowl.

2. Whisk together the lime juice, olive oil, salt, black pepper, garlic, and cayenne pepper and pour over the vegetables.

3. Toss well.

4. Just before you're ready to serve the salad, fold the avocados into the salad.

5. Check the seasoning and serve at room temperature.

Trinity Fitness
By Jackson John-Maire

Greek Tomato Salad

Ingredients

- 4.0 fresh tomatoes chopped
- 1.0 cucumbers peeled and chopped
- 1.0 green bell peppers cut into 1/2 ",pieces
- 0.5 cups red onions
- 1.0 tablespoons vinegar
- 1.0 tablespoons vinegar
- 1.0 tablespoons extra virgin olive oil
- 1.0 teaspoons salt
- 1.0 tablespoons fresh oregano
- 0.25 cups kalamata olives
- 0.5 cups feta cheese crumbled I use the fat free type

Directions

1. Mix together vinegars, oil, salt and oregano.

2. Add other ingredients.

3. Marinate several hours in refrigerator to allow flavors to blend.

4. Serve.

Trinity Fitness

By Jackson John-Maire

Dinner

Easy Broccoli Soup

Ingredients

- 1.0 tablespoons oil
- 1.0 onions diced
- 2.0 garlic cloves minced or use 2 teasp from a jar
- 1.0 large head broccoli trimmed and chopped, about 500g
- 1.0 potatoes peeled & diced or leave skin on if you prefer
- 6.0 cups chicken stock homemade, from a carton or use 6 teasp granules to 6 cups water or to your taste
- 1.0 to taste salt & freshly ground black pepper
- 2.0 slices bacon diced, optional variation

Directions

1. In a large deep pan heat the oil over medium and add the onion & garlic.

2. Cook gently until softened for about 2-3 minutes.

3. Add the potato, broccoli and stock and bring to the boil.

4. Turn heat down and simmer for 20 mins until vegetables are cooked.

5. Either pour into a blender and blend or use a stick blender in pan to make a smooth mixture.

6. If using a blender add soup back to the pan and heat gently.

7. It is at this point you can add the chopped bacon and simmer til bacon is cooked, about 15mins, then check seasoning.

8. If not adding the bacon, check seasoning and add salt & pepper to taste & reheat gently.

9. Serve in nice bowls with slices of french bread which have been toasted on one side, turned over and topped with either blue cheese or whatever cheese you have on hand and grilled for a few mins til melted & crispy, on the side.

Ww Herbed Spilt Pea Soup

Ingredients

- 2.0 teaspoons olive oil
- 1.0 onions chopped
- 2.0 carrots peeled and chopped
- 2.0 garlic cloves minced
- 1.0 cups dried split peas rinsed
- 14.5 ounces vegetable broth
- 2.0 cups water
- 0.5 cups ham slivered
- 1.0 teaspoons dried marjoram
- 0.125 teaspoons salt
- 0.125 teaspoons pepper

Directions

1. Heat the oil in a saucepan, saute the onion, carrot, and garlic until softened 5 minutes.

2. Add the split peas water and broth, and bring to a boil. Cover, reduce the heat and simmer until the peas are tender, approxiamtely 1 hour.

3. Stir in the remaining ingredients.

Trinity Fitness
By Jackson John-Maire

Low-Fat Cream of Chicken and Wild Rice Soup

Ingredients

- 1.0 lbs boneless skinless chicken breasts diced into 1/2 to 1/4 chunks
- 1.0 medium onions diced
- 1.0 cups baby carrots
- 0.5 cups celery
- 2.0 cups cooked wild rice
- 5.0 cups fat-free chicken broth or less if you want it thicker
- 1.0 cups fat-free half-and-half
- 3.0 tablespoons flour
- 1.0 tablespoons reduced fat margarine
- 2.0 tablespoons dry sherry
- 0.25 teaspoons salt
- 0.25 teaspoons pepper
- 0.5 teaspoons thyme

Directions

1. In a large stock pot, sauté chicken until cooked through. Remove to a bowl. Add wild rice to the bowl. Mix in the half and half, sherry, and flour. Set aside.

2. In the same pot, melt butter. Cook onion until soft and translucent. Add carrots and celery, salt, pepper, and thyme. Cook, stirring, for about 5 minutes.

3. Add chicken broth. Bring to a boil, reduce heat, cover and simmer for about 15 minutes, or until carrots and celery are softened to your liking.

4. Stir in the wild rice and chicken mixture. Cook, stirring, for about 5 minutes, until heated through.

Trinity Fitness
By Jackson John-Maire

Lemon Pepper Fish Greek Style

Ingredients

- 2.0 garlic cloves crushed
- 0.25 cups olive oil
- 1.0 tablespoons lemon juice
- 0.5 teaspoons lemon zest finely zested
- 0.5 teaspoons cracked black pepper
- 0.5 teaspoons sea salt
- 1.0 teaspoons dried oregano leaves
- 2.0 fish fillets 1 pound/1/2 kilo estimate

Directions

1. Combine the garlic, oil, lemon juice, lemon zest, cracked black pepper, sea salt and the dried oregano in a large bowl. Use the bowl in which you will marinate your fish.

2. Add the fish and ensure it is thoroughly coated in the marinade. Cover and refrigerate for 15-20 minutes.

3. Line a broiler/griller tray with aluminium foil and place the fish on in a single layer. Broil/Grill the fish for 5-10 minutes each side. Only turn the fish once during the cooking (as you do not want it to fall apart). Grill until the fish is cooked.

4. Serve with a salad or veges.

Sweet Potato Buffalo Fries

Ingredients

- 4.0 sweet potatoes
- 3.0 tablespoons olive oil
- 0.125 teaspoons chili powder
- 0.125 teaspoons cayenne
- 0.125 teaspoons garlic salt

Directions

1. Preheat oven to 425°F.

2. Peel and slice potatoes into 1 inch wedges.

3. Toss with oil.

4. Mix together seasonings, sprinkle over potatoes and toss to coat.

5. Place on a baking sheet and roast 30 minutes, turning often, until golden.

6. Sprinkle with salt if desired.

Trinity Fitness
By Jackson John-Maire

Easy, Healthy Baked Chicken Breasts

Ingredients

- 8.0 ounces boneless skinless chicken breasts
- 0.5 cups chicken broth
- 0.25 teaspoons onion powder
- 0.25 teaspoons garlic salt
- 1.0 to taste fresh ground black pepper

Directions

1. Preheat oven to 350 degrees.

2. Rinse, and pat chicken breasts dry. Spray small, shallow baking dish with cooking spray. Sprinkle chicken with onion powder, garlic salt, and pepper. Place in baking dish. Add chicken broth to dish.

3. Bake 20 minutes or until no longer pink.

Healthy Sesame Chicken

Ingredients

- 0.25 cups unbleached flour
- 0.25 cups all-purpose flour
- 0.25 teaspoons salt
- 0.125 teaspoons ground black pepper
- 4.0 boneless skinless chicken breast halves cut into 2 inch 4 inch strips
- 0.25 cups reduced sodium soy sauce
- 0.25 cups sugar
- 0.5 teaspoons dark sesame oil
- 2.0 tablespoons sesame seeds toasted
- 0.25 cups fresh chives

Directions

1. In a gallon-size plastic bag, combine flour, salt and pepper.

2. Add chicken, seal bag, and shake well to coat.

3. Coat a large nonstick skillet with nonstick spray and warm over medium-high heat.

4. Add chicken to skillet and cook, stirring, for 3 to 4 minutes, or until no longer pink.

5. Transfer to a plate.

6. Reduce heat to medium.

7. Combine soy sauce and sugar in the skillet.

8. Cook, stirring occasionally, until the sugar dissolves.

9. Add oil and sesame seeds.

Trinity Fitness
By Jackson John-Maire

Easy Chicken & Potato Dinner

Ingredients

- 2.0 lbs chicken breasts bone-in
- 2.0 lbs chicken thighs bone-in
- 1.0 lbs potatoes cut into wedges
- 4.0 small carrots cut into small chunks
- 0.5 cups Italian dressing
- 1.0 tablespoons italian seasoning
- 0.5 cups parmesan cheese

Directions

1. Place chicken, potato& carrot in 13" X 9" dish.

2. Pour dressing over dish contents.

3. Sprinkle with seasonings and parmesan cheese.

4. Bake, uncovered, at 400 for 1 hour or until chicken is cooked through.

Trinity Fitness
By Jackson John-Maire

Healthy Chicken/Turkey Burgers

Ingredients

- 1.0 lbs ground chicken
- 1.0 lbs ground turkey
- 0.5 cups plain breadcrumbs
- 0.25 cups applesauce
- 0.25 cups yellow onions minced
- 0.25 cups parsley chopped
- 1.0 teaspoons Worcestershire sauce
- 1.0 teaspoons lemon juice
- 1.0 to taste salt and pepper

Directions

1. Combine all ingredients and shape into patties.

2. Grill, broil or saute about 4 to 5 minutes per side.

Trinity Fitness
By Jackson John-Maire

Healthy Sloppy Joes

Ingredients

- 0.5 cups onions chopped
- 1.0 garlic cloves minced
- 10.0 ounces ground turkey
- 0.5 cups canned black beans rinsed
- 1.0 cups tomato puree
- 1.0 tablespoons cider vinegar
- 1.0 teaspoons chili powder
- 0.25 teaspoons mustard powder
- 8.0 whole wheat dinner rolls

Directions

1. Lightly coat a medium skillet with cooking spray and heat over medium-high. Add onion and garlic and cook until onion softens, about 5 minutes.

2. Add ground turkey and cook, stirring to break up the meat. Cook until no longer pink, about 5 minutes.

3. Stir in remaining ingredients (except dinner rolls!). Cook until bubbly and slightly thickened. Divide evenly over dinner rolls and serve hot.

Trinity Fitness
By Jackson John-Maire

Healthy Waldorf Turkey Salad Sandwiches

Ingredients

- 1.0 cups cooked turkey
- 0.667 cups apples
- 1.0 celery ribs finely chopped
- 0.5 cups walnuts toasted
- 0.25 cups golden raisins
- 0.333 cups non-fat vanilla yogurt
- 0.333 cups fat-free mayonnaise
- 0.5 teaspoons dried tarragon
- 0.5 teaspoons orange peel
- 0.125 teaspoons kosher salt
- 1.0 dashes fresh ground pepper
- 4.0 sandwich buns split

Directions

1. In a bowl, combine the turkey, apple, celery, walnuts and raisins.

2. In a separate small bowl, combine the yogurt, mayonnaise, tarragon, orange peel, salt and pepper.

3. Pour dressing over turkey mixture and stir to coat. Spoon 1/2 cup onto each roll.

Healthy Black Bean Soup With Turkey Sausage

Ingredients

- 6.0 ounces turkey sausage sliced
- 1.0 red bell peppers diced
- 15.0 ounces chicken broth fat free
- 15.0 ounces black beans rinsed and drained
- 15.0 ounces tomatoes diced
- 0.25 cups red onions diced
- 1.0 garlic cloves minced
- 1.0 chipotle peppers minced
- 0.25 teaspoons cumin
- 1.0 to taste salt
- 1.0 to taste pepper

Directions

1. Spray a soup pan with cooking spray and bring up to medium high heat. Add onions and cook for about 2 minutes. Add the sausage and cook for another two minutes. Add the bell pepper and garlic. Cook an additional 2 minutes.

2. Add the broth, cumin, and tomatoes. Bring to a boil. Reduce the heat to a simmer and add chipotle and beans. Cook covered for about 10 minutes.

3. Season to taste with salt and pepper.

4. Serve with a sprinkle of Cilantro or some fat free sour cream.

5. **Variation Idea: I have tried this as a smooth soup -- brown off the turkey in a separate pan, following all of the other directions up until the point the beans are added. I use a hand held blender to blend up the soup. Afterwards I add the turkey and some additional beans to give a little texture.

Healthy Fish Sticks

Ingredients

- 2.0 white fish fillets cut into strips i've used cod and sole
- 0.667 cups oatmeal
- 3.0 tablespoons dried parsley
- 1.0 tablespoons garlic powder
- 1.0 tablespoons onion powder
- 1.0 to taste salt
- 1.0 to taste pepper
- 1.0 egg whites
- 2.0 tablespoons olive oil to grease pan, drizzle on top

Directions

1. Preheat oven to 450°F.

2. Line a cookie sheet with tin foil and grease with 1 tablespoon of olive oil.

3. Mix oatmeal, parsley, garlic and onion powder, salt and pepper in a medium sized bowl.

4. In a separate bowl, beat the egg white slightly.

5. Dip strips of fish in the egg white then transfer to oatmeal mixture bowl and cover strip completely with oatmeal mixture and place on cookie sheet.

6. Drizzle remaining olive oil on top of strips.

7. Bake for 15 minutes, flipping half way through.

Trinity Fitness

By Jackson John-Maire

Grocery List Ideas and Recommendation

1. Bakery and Bread

On Your List:

1. Whole wheat bread, pita pockets, and English muffins
2. Whole-grain flour tortillas

Look for the words "whole wheat" or "whole wheat flour" as the first ingredient on the label.

Choose whole-grain breads that contain at least 3 to 4 grams of fiber and have fewer than 100 calories per slice.

2. Meat and Seafood

On Your List:

1. Skinless chicken or turkey breasts
2. Ground turkey or chicken
3. Salmon, halibut, trout, mackerel
4. Reduced-sodium lunchmeat (turkey, roast beef)

If you buy red meat, choose the leanest cuts -- ones with very little marbling.

Eat ground chicken or ground turkey breast instead of ground beef. These are much lower in fat. Get creative with the condiments and you'll get flavor without the fat.

3. Pasta and Rice

On Your List:

1. Brown rice
2. Whole wheat or whole-grain pasta

Again, favor whole grains whenever possible.

4. Oils, Sauces, Salad Dressings, and Condiments

On Your List:

1. Tomato sauce
2. Mustard
3. Barbecue sauce
4. Red-wine vinegar
5. Salsa
6. Extra virgin olive oil or canola oil, nonfat cooking spray
7. Jarred capers and olives
8. Hot pepper sauce

Many sauces and condiments are surprisingly high in sodium and sugar. Look for sugar-free varieties. Keep track of sodium levels, especially if you're cutting back on salt.

Replace mayonnaise and other high-fat condiments with fat-free options like salsa and hot sauce.

5. Cereals and Breakfast Foods

On Your List:

1. Whole-grain or multigrain cereals
2. Steel-cut or instant oatmeal
3. Whole-grain cereal bars

Buy cereals and cereal bars that are high in fiber and low in sugar. Use berries, dried fruit, or nuts to add sweetness to your cereal.